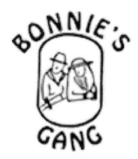

Bonnie's Gang Publishing

is proud to present:

D1546536

Go to:

BonniesGang.com

Sign-up for our newsletter,

and receive your bonus report:

Hot and Heavy

Top Five Myths about the Female Orgasm

The sixth book in the "Sex Made Easy" series:

Boink Her Pink:

The Ultimate Guide to the G-spot Orgasm

G-gasm.com

G-gasm Method for Lesbian Lovers:

G-spot Orgasm Secrets Revealed

BonnieGang.com

Tonight's the Night: Ultimate Guide to Sexy, Kinky Things to do With Your Lover

BonniesGang.com

BlowPons ... Blowjob Coupons

BlowPons.com

Why Women Love Cavemen –

A Man's Guide to Tame the Bitch

WomenTamed.com

Got Milked?

Prostate Massage for Prostate Health & Sexual Fulfillment

Your Ultimate Guide to Milk Your Man's Penis

Got Milked?

Published by Bonnie's Gang Publishing 2009, New York

Although based on actual experience, some events in this book have been fictionalized to protect the privacy of certain individuals.

Please consult your doctor if you have any kind of a medical condition involving the prostate, anus or penis before using the P-gasm Method. As with anything, use common sense.

While a prostate massage can be of some benefit, it is important to be aware that there are risks involved with massaging a prostate that is suffering from an ailment or using too much force through the rectum wall. Use minimum pressure and reasonable vigor, or damage to the very sensitive soft tissues and nerves may occur.

Bonnie's Gang Publishing

Please visit us at: BonniesGang.com

ISBN # 0-9762090-7-1

For the all the woman that have experienced
G-gasms, who wish to reciprocate.

CONTENTS

INTRODUCTION

I watched intently as Andrea removed her pantyhose and teasingly she trailed them over my face. I grabbed the nylons as the toes were dangling right in front of me and placed the crotch directly over my nose, my heart was racing, "ahh … that smells so delicious better than cotton candy." Andrea's pantyhose smelled just like her, a slight hint of perfume and the sweet smell of her sex.

I was lying down on the bed, my head propped against the wall against a fluffy pillow. Andrea sat on the bed next to me. She was not overly attractive, but had tits to die for. I had not seen Andrea for quite some time. She had taken to dying her hair auburn brown, a serious change from its former blonde state. She had a series of very light brown freckles that ran from under her eyes on one cheek, over her nose and onto her other cheek. We had just returned to my place, fresh from a night of club-hopping.

I knew Andrea since my first year in college. She would call me up and ask, "Hey, you want to go smoke a joint?"

I knew it and she knew it – she might as well asked me if I felt like getting together, party and have sex. That was her code, her MO when she felt horny. Andrea was a lot of fun; more often than not, except if I had something better going,

I would say okay and meet with her.

Andrea leaned over to kiss me. We had kissed passionately on numerous occasions, but I didn't want Andrea to get the wrong idea. I liked her, but I didn't love her – she was my FB – fuck buddy. She lay down next to me; her legs intertwined with mine, as I put my hands on her hips and rubbed her butt, our sets of lips met and I gently nibbled her tongue. We kissed long and hard, kisses that explored each other's mouth – her kisses tasted differently tonight - almost like spicy vanilla.

Andrea straddled my hips, sat up and removed my shirt. From this position, I got the best view of those beautiful tits. I think she loved those hooters just as much as I did. She put one of her hands on her pussy, pleasuring herself gently while whispering in my ear that her tits were better, bigger and firmer than Britney's or Paris's

In reality, her tits were not big; it was the shape and configuration that made them outstanding. Perfect. Not too big, not too small, big enough to play with but nothing wasted. And, after some of the girls I've been with lately (you know the ones with the silicone implants), her tits are not phony, they are warm and squishy, I hate it when girls try to fake it.

My cock, now as hard as a hunting rifle aimed at an unsuspecting deer, was standing straight up in the air. Andrea, looked me up and down,

12

her gaze lingered where my cock grazed against her hot crotch. My cock, straining against the layers of clothing that separates me from Andrea's pussy. "That looks so hot and tasty," Andrea managed to say.

Andrea slid down my legs her pussy now nestled against the top of my feet; she leaned over unbuttoned and unzipped my jeans. I hardly ever wear underwear, so Andrea had easy access to my now hard as concrete cock. After a bit of pulling and maneuvering, my cock was in her mouth. Before I knew it, the head of my cock was firmly lodged in Andrea's throat. Andrea sucked with greed and enthusiasm, playing with me like I was her private little toy.

"The best five minutes of silence that any man can experience," I thought to myself.

Andrea is a serious cocksucker – here are a few of her tips for you ladies:

TIPS ON HOW TO GIVE A GREAT BLOW JOB:

Giving a blowjob is an adventure, not a chore, but a pleasurable thing for both the giver and receiver.

All men might be created equal, but all men like their monkey handled in different ways. Don't assume you know what he likes – experiment, talk or follow his leads. Don't think your mouth has to do it all by itself, use

13

your hands for assistance and variation.

Gals, be sure to pay attention to the whole penis, not just the head. Swirl your tongue around the head while pumping him with your hand.

For many men, hummers are a visual experience – make sure he can watch. A strategically placed mirror can be a huge turn-on for him.

If your jaw gets a little tired, don't be afraid to hop on him and ride him for a few minutes, before going back down to finish the job. I guarantee the thought of you tasting your sweet love juices on his favorite tool will add to his excitement.

If your man is a challenge to get to the finish line make sure he's good and turned on before you start. Get him half way there before you start by watching some porn, flirting or while on a date whisper in his ear you aren't wearing any panties.

Don't forget the twins below. Lovingly massage his balls and sack – the heat from your lips and tongue gives him an amazing sensation.

Deep throat. This may cause some gagging and welling of tears, but you must learn to suck it up and take it.

When you are in the down position on the deep throat, gently nod your head up and down and side to side and make a little humming noise – guaranteed to drive him wild – they are called hummers for a reason.

Alternate your speed and tempo when sucking his cock.

Repeat this process as often as necessary to complete the job. The job is done when the man shoots his hot, thick load down your throat, at which point, you should swallow with relish and joy. This too, may cause some gagging, resulting in some of the load to be spewed out of the corner of your mouth, but learn to enjoy the experience.

When he does start to come   don't stop what you are doing, suck until he is finished.

Spit, swallow or point and shoot? Always swallow with a smile : o), but that's me speaking, I am a man. Andrea always loved to swallow, but the choice is yours – at the very least, try it you might like it.

I have never seen a survey on the topic, but I would guess that most men don't care all that much what you do with his love juices. I can think of one girl in particular that always used the "point and shoot" technique. She would remove her lips just seconds before I climaxed and stroked me until I had a puddle of cum on my stomach.

ANDREA'S BLOW JOB SURPRISE

My cock, hard enough to cut a diamond, was ready for action.

"I have a big surprise for you tonight," Andrea whispered sheepishly.

"What? A surprise? What the hell – what Andrea was doing to me right now was pure paradise – you mean it gets better?" I thought to myself. I was in a state of euphoria now with Andrea dedicating her very talented skills to eating my fully enlarged cock. "What could she possibly do to make things better?"

Andrea moved her lips near mine. "That felt so good," I told Andrea softly. We kissed, and although I have often kissed her with the taste of her pussy in my mouth, the taste and scent of my cock was very titillating. With my arms around her soft shoulders, I pulled her closer to me and kissed her deeply.

I was hot and ready, my raging hard-on throbbing with anticipation of release. Andrea got that look in her eyes that I know so well. She had a wicked little smile on her face that said,

"Wait 'till you see what I have in store for you."

Andrea let out a little giggle, "There is an area of you that I have never before explored."

"What the hell is she talking about," I thought to myself with my little heart pounding, "what is she thinking?"

"We have never played that milking thing that I heard about," Andrea said matter-of-factly.

"What is this milking thingie you're talking about," I ask, my curiosity piqued.

"It is something I read about on the Internet – a new way to pleasure your man," Andrea replied, "Lay back, enjoy and follow my instructions."

Not one to argue ...

GETTING STARTED

Guys and gals, you are about to learn a life changing sex method. Sex will never be as it once was. Ladies, once you master this, he will be your sex slave forever.

First off, I am not a celebrity or a sex therapist. I am not a doctor so this book will not provide you with any form of medical jargon. You will not find a flow chart of the vagina, penis, anus or any type of medical advice that you could logically expect to find when you are speaking to a doctor. If you are looking for that kind of information, I am sorry, Yahoo "female vagina," "male penis," or whatever technical information you are looking for – you will get all the info you need. There is not a doctor in the world that will teach you, what you are about to learn here.

I have never really kept track, but I have made love to (done, fucked, screwed ... whatever) over 50 women. I have no medical training but I can teach you plenty of things about a man's body, his P-spot and the right way to stimulate it to create mind blowing orgasms. The P-gasm Method is not hard to do once you know exactly where to find the P-spot, and how to fire it up correctly.

After my best selling book "Boink Her Pink" AKA "The G-gasm Method" took to the shelves, the biggest question that I get from the ladies is

"How do I return the favor – how do I return the favor and reciprocate?"

Well, here it is – "Got Milked" AKA "The P-gasm Method."

WHAT IS THE P-SPOT OR MALE G-SPOT?

The P-spot is the sexual equivalent of the G-spot in females. We all know about the clitoris, the exposed part of the female sex plumbing, and now after reading the G-gasm Method we know about the G-spot and its function during sex.

A QUICK RECAP OF THE G-SPOT AND THE G-GASM METHOD

The G-spot is located about 2-3 inches inside the vagina on the outside or anterior wall. That is it – no mystery, no nothing – that is the G-spot. It is not like the lost city of Atlantis or some beautiful, secret area run by the CIA.

You can imagine your partner's G-spot as almost opposite her clitoris but below the surface on the inside anterior wall of her vagina.

When you have felt your way around in the vagina, you'll get to know the G-spot, as "bump" surrounded by the smooth fleshy anterior wall. The "bump" will feel ribbed, almost like the roof of your mouth. Memorize

19

the first sentence of this paragraph.

Direct G-spot stimulation manually, either with your fingers or a toy or with a penis, produces waves of G-gasms AKA G-spot orgasms.

Recent discoveries about the size of the clitoris - it extends inside the body - would seem to support my theory about G-gasms. The nerves of the clitoris pass through the G-spot and connect to the spinal cord for transmission to the brain cells. As the G-spot is stimulated, it grows in size.

In technical terms, the G-spot is a bundle of nerve clusters that trigger natural painkillers within a woman's body. These painkillers are the same endorphins that release during childbirth. The nerve endings are concentrated beneath the surface of the skin in a protective bundle, which allows for sensitivity and ability to handle fondling.

An un-stimulated G-spot is only about the size of a pea and feels kind of like a dry roasted peanut shell. As the G-spot gets aroused and stimulated it swells to the size of a small walnut, giving you the clue that you not only found the spot but that it likes you.

The G-gasm Method is all about "waking up" the G-spot to make her explode with pleasure.

WHERE IS THE P-SPOT OR MALE G-SPOT?

The p-spot in a man is the sexual aspect of the prostate gland. The main function of the prostate is to store and secrete a clear fluid that accounts for up to one-third of the volume of semen. Semen is composed of spermatozoa and seminal fluid, some produced by the prostate gland, the rest is produced by the two seminal vesicles. This fluid provides nutritional energy for the brave sperm as they swim up the female reproductive system and try to fertilize the egg.

The prostate also contains smooth muscles that contract during ejaculation to expel the fluid.

That is as technical as I get here – if you want more information about the male or female reproductive system you can easily look it up – in this book, we are concerned about the pleasure aspect of the p-spot.

The p-spot is NOT in the anus. It can be stimulated through the rectum wall, but it lies below the bladder and next to the rectum. If the man is lying on his back, with you between his legs, finger inserted palm side up do a "come here" motion, towards his penis, you will feel a chestnut sized mound - **that is the p-spot**.

The p -spot feels like a firm bulge about the size of a walnut. Be gentle, and as with anything take your cues from your mans reactions. He will let you know by his movements and body positioning what he wants.

Guys, I recommend you experiment and explore your body. Learn where your p-spot is before you let your lover explore. This way you can advise her (or him) where the spot is and what to do with it. Not finding the spot and not knowing what to do with it can lead to frustration and disappointment.

While squatting, or standing with one leg propped up on a chair or any firm surface, place one well-lubed finger in your anus from between your thighs. You need to be flexible and have long enough arms. Short stubby fingers might also be a problem. You also have to have enough courage to do it. It is somewhat frightening the first time but gets to be routine after some practice. Get yourself in a sexually excited state before you go probing around for the p-spot. Feel around outwards, or towards the front for something that feels good when you press it – that is the p-spot.

Another method is to lie down on your bed on your left side (if right handed) and try to work your index finger into position. Start by bringing your right knee up towards your chest and then straightening up after entry. The hand goes behind your back, not through your legs. With a well-lubed finger, start by massaging the opening and then gently insert your finger in your anus.

Either way, the angle is awkward - you might want to experiment with a long thin dildo – one that preferably has a slight bend in the top. Ask your wife or girlfriend if you can borrow theirs for "research." Maybe that is not a good idea ... prostate massagers are available on the Internet – go to P-Gasm.com - do a search for "prostate massager."

Unless you are a contortionist, you will not be able to experience p-gasms by your self – because of your angle of entry, steady pressure is hard to maintain. You will be able to find your p-spot. You want to know where your p-spot is located and the feelings when stimulated. With a FB working your p-spot, you do not have to worry. Your FB can keep going long after you are looking like a pretzel and are unable to continue because of complete fatigue.

WHAT IS A P-GASM?

P-gasms are orgasms enhanced by prostate massage or prostate milking. "Massage" or "milking" are generally interchangeable, although in our discussions we are talking about something done in a sexual nature – not for physical therapy, medical procedure or anything like that. P-gasms are much more intense and longer lasting than a regular orgasm.

Remember that all men are different – down to our sexual plumbing, so each mans reactions will be different. Some men report that a P-gasm seems like an orgasm in slow motion – one that lasts for a minute or more. Most guys will ooze an abnormal amount of precum – to the point of "Holy shit I won't have anything left for an orgasm" but then when they do explode they cum in "ropes." Some guys report a side-effect that they have an urge for another orgasm within minutes of a prostate stimulated orgasm.

There are many variations to P-gasms. There is no one answer – it depends on your plumbing and how the prostate is stimulated. One thing for sure – a P-gasm is much more intense and more of a full body experience.

PREPARING FOR A PROSTATE MILKING

While a prostate massage can be of some benefit, it is important to be aware that there are risks involved with massaging a prostate that is suffering from an ailment or using too much force.

Use minimum pressure and use reasonable vigor, or damage to the very sensitive soft tissues and nerves may occur. Remember, those are real membranes and tissue up there in that dark cave – it is easy to be carried away with the sensations. Use common sense.

Most of the online sex toyshops sell a version of a "Prostate Massager." For privacy, go to one of the online stores such as adamandeve.com or sextoy.com. Do a search for "prostate" and you'll have many choices to choose from. Generally, these toys are similar to a finger, because a finger is the best way to milk a man. Use a massager with care, in that the prostate and the anus region in general are sensitive. Do not use in a thrusting manner – massage gently in a circular, side-to-side or back and forth motion.

By far the best way to properly milk a man is with your finger(s). Prepare your hands for this erotic experience. Scrub your hands well. Long manicured fingernails may look good, but not for what you are about to do. Keep the nails short and filed smooth. NO FAKE NAILS – many hospitals and doctors offices have banned the use of fake fingernails in the work area. Apparently, there is some doubt as to the cleanliness of the area beneath the fake nails. But more importantly, you don't want to lose one of your fake nails while buried deep in his man-hole. Why take a chance?

Before you begin the activities, to help prevent rough, dry hands in any weather, be sure to routinely massage your favorite hand cream thoroughly into your hands. The massaging action stimulates blood circulation throughout the hands and promotes the absorption of conditioners into your skin. Apply your favorite hand cream often, especially after

25

washing your hands or after submerging them in water. Your lover will really appreciate your prep work.

For those that want a little "protection" there are a variety of products named "Finger Gloves," "Finger Cots," "Finger Caps" etc. that provide a thin layer of protection between your finger and Honey's butt hole. Do an Internet search for any of the above words and you will easily find them. Wal-Mart or any of the big drug stores carry them also.

DON'T FORGET THE LUBE! Chances are that you are entering a virgin butt hole – you need plenty of lube. I have found that water based lubricants are best. Just about any of the commercial name brands are fine. In an emergency i.e. "not prepared" you can use baby oil, mineral oil, Vaseline petroleum jelly, and even cooking oils are safe. Lately, sweetie and I are experimenting with pure virgin coconut oil. Turns out, coconut oil is excellent for the skin, is easily absorbed and possesses great healing properties.

Never use an oil-based lube with a condom — it will cause it to weaken and break.

Avoid using soap or shampoo as a lube as they can be irritants and can cause skin and membranes dryness and irritation. I have received numerous "please help" e-mails from guys whose skin has suddenly turned leathery and cracked, or the skin has begun massively peeling. Although it eventually heals, it can be scary.

Again, I am not a doctor, but as I mentioned earlier, coconut oil is has healing affects on the skin. Go to a doctor if you are having unpleasant skin conditions, but in the mean time, rubbing on some coconut oil can't hurt.

GET OVER THE HOMOPHOBIA EFFECT

A big problem for some men is that they will feel like less of a man if they let someone play with their ass. GET OVER IT! Seriously, guys, you do not want to pass this up – The P-gasm Method opens up a new area that needs exploration. I have received notes and e-mails from wives complaining about not being able to try The Method because of hubby's attitude about anal play.

Yeah right, just because your wife or girlfriend sticks a finger up your ass while blowing you is NOT going to turn you into a flaming fag. That's just stupid.

If another guy was playing and fondling your butt, I would say that you are gay, or at least bi-sexual. Guys, look next to you – does that person have tits and NO COCK? If the answer is "yes" and "yes" – then you are NOT engaging in any homosexual acts. Relax, let her play and have fun.

Some husbands / boyfriends are afraid to try the method because of the fear of the unknown – their inhibitions are mainly from lack of experience rather than homophobia. What you ladies have to do is – accidentally leave this book in the bathroom; we all know men do their best reading there. Remember also, bondage does come in handy.

THE P-GASM METHOD

OK, does everybody know where the p-spot is?

One more time – everybody together: The p-spot is NOT in the anus. It is stimulated through the rectum wall, but it lies below the bladder and next to the rectum. If the man is lying on his back, with you between his legs, finger inserted palm side up do a "come here" motion, towards his penis, you will feel a chestnut sized mound - the p-spot. Thank you! Very good - let's party!

Now that we all know where the p-spot is – it is time to have some fun. The most important thing you can remember is that every man is different. No man has the same attitude towards this type of play. Take it easy – relax, have fun and make it fun for your partner. Communication is key, encourage him to talk but also you need to learn how to read his body language.

The P-gasm Method is all about the woman stimulating the prostate as a means of inducing an intense, heightened massive quantity orgasm or as a means of extending the time and length of the orgasm or a combination of both.

Anal play can be painful especially for virgin

butts, if done properly it will be pure pleasure. Pain anywhere in the body is a sign that something is wrong, same with the anal area. There is an abundance of nerve endings in the anal area that can produce enormous pain if mistreated, or extraordinary enjoyment if done properly.

When an object is inserted into the anus, whether it is a finger or a dildo, the anal sphincter muscles want to lock up to stop the intrusion. Do not force anything into the anus until these muscles are relaxed, or extreme pain can develop. If he says "no," he probably means it – he needs to relax more.

Deep breathing and tensing the sphincter muscles then relaxing them will help him loosen up, but probably the best way to introduce anal play is in a hot shower or bath. After promising not to penetrate him, play with his ass to let him become more familiar with the wonderful sensations while learning to relax.

Do not overlook the psychological aspect of anal play. For some men, the "taboo" of someone playing with their ass adds a special thrill. Other men develop a frown on their face and consider their anus a secret, special area – not a toy.

Rimming (oral sex in the anal area) is considered either disgusting, disgustingly sleazy, or delightfully perverse. Most people either love it or hate it – the two of you can decide.

By no means should anyone attempt any anal penetration if there is anything physically wrong with the rectum, prostate, bladder area. Guys, never tolerate physical pain, it can cause injury. Gals, never use force and both of you avoid or limit the use of drugs and alcohol as they can cloud clear thinking and actions. Be wary of STD's and keep up with your hygiene – other than that, let's have some fun and party.

Later on, we will discuss variations of the basic P-gasm Method. Some of these variations will work better for you than others and will bring different results with various men. Some men will not have any huge orgasms but they may enjoy the intimacy and still receive enormous pleasure. Again, it just depends on the man. Either way, plan to spend the first evening exploring his body.

BACK TO ANDREA

Andrea, sitting cross-legged between my outstretched legs, pulled her hair back over her shoulders, and grabbed hold of my hard cock. She fondled me ever so gently and with her other hand she moved my legs over her thighs. With my legs over her thighs, Andrea now was able to slide closer in to my crotch. She continued to stroke my shaft, causing me to let out a soft moan.

Andrea leaned over to the bed table, opened the draw and took out a bottle of Slip 'n Slide. She applied a generous amount over my cock, and wrapped her long thin fingers around my shaft.

She smiled, "Ooo … that's better, I like the slippery feel," as she smacked and spanked my cock around a bit."

After a few more strokes, she began to rub her thumb very slowly up and down my pole and along the sensitive head of my cock. She finished each slow torturous thumb rub by squeezing the head of my cock firmly between her fingers. My body tensed up and I raise my hips into the air. She saw what her thumb rubbing was doing to me and smiled fiendishly at me.

"You like it when I do that with my fingers – don't you," Andrea asked knowing she needed no response, "well, you are really going to like what I do with my fingers later."

I let out a little moan every time Andrea's slippery fingers passed over the head of my cock. Soon I leaked some precum as Andrea watched it ooze out of my slit and dribble over her thumb. Andrea giggled, "Amazing what my fingers can do." My cock now throbbing in her hand, "I love that."

Andrea stopped what she was doing, and began to fondle with my **balls. She moved her fingers to the area between my sack and my butt.**

With her index and middle finger, gently, yet firmly Andrea applied pressure to the taint area. I wasn't sure, but it kind of felt good – sent a chill and shiver up my spine.

"Do you like that," Andrea whispered.

"Yeah baby that feels good," I replied as Andrea moved her fingers south and let them rest on top of my butt hole.

"Could this be what she was talking about before about the 'unexplored areas' that needed servicing," I thought to myself. "Was she really going to go in there??!! Oh my god!" Andrea reached over and mounded some more Slip 'n Slide on her fingers.

Andrea reached back down, and gently bounced her fingers on my ass hole. "I can't believe I'm about to lose my virginity down there, but it felt surprisingly good," I thought to myself. Andrea traced the hole with her fingers. "Ahhh … that felt nice …" I was actually aching for her to stick a finger in my ass.

Her finger traced around my ass one more time, then she plunged her finger into my hole. "Holy shit," I yelled! I felt every inch of that finger in my asshole – it was an amazing feeling –I wasn't sure if I was supposed to like it, but I did. It took a while for my tight, virgin hole to loosen up. I tried to relax my ass as much as possible.

'Relax Honey; you are safe. I'm going to move

my finger around a bit so that you get used to it."
I felt Andrea's finger move up and down and around inside me.

'Is that it?" I asked.

"Oh no Sweetie, I am just warming you up." As I started feeling more relaxed, Andrea pushed her finger in all the way. 'Just relax and accept me." Andrea moved her finger a little more and said, "Almost there now."

I relaxed a little and soon the odd feeling of her finger in my rectum started to actually feel good. I cried out in encouragement, "Wow that feels so good - I love that feeling!" By now, my cock is twitching and throbbing – with a big wad of precum oozing out.

Suddenly, by moving her finger Andrea hit a new spot, "Oh my God," I groaned loudly.

"Oh, I poked something inside you that has never been touched before," Andrea said. "I'm all the way in – how does it feel when I probe around your p-spot?"

"That's wonderful," I managed to blurt out. Every time she touched the spot, is a sent tingly buzzing feeling down my legs to my toes and through my balls to the tip of my cock.

"Now the fun begins. I want you to remain relaxed and put your knees up in the air a bit." Andrea moved in closer to me, her head inches from the bulging red head of my dick. "Let the milking begin."

"What? What the hell is she talking about – Milking?" I tried to visualize what she was doing to me and how she was going to milk my cock.

Andrea grabbed my cock with her free hand; the other remained firmly nestled in my ass against my p-spot. She licked the growing mound of precum delicately balanced at the tip of my cock before it streamed down the shaft. "Mmmm …. tasty. Oh my God, you are leaking like crazy already. That's HOT!"

Andrea kept my solidified cock firmly between her fingers. She moved her hand down to the base, then slowly, yet forcefully towards the swollen head. Her other hand is slowly pumping my ass, hitting my p-spot repeatedly. I felt so violated, yet it felt amazing. Every time she hit the spot, my cock undulated backwards towards my stomach. "Holy crap … that feels unbelievable!" All of a sudden, I felt a new feeling as Andrea inserted another finger.

Gradually she increased the speed of her thrusts, her mouth now full of my red meat. Andrea, slurping and sucking as hard as she could had a hard time eating all the oozing cum. She took her mouth off, I propped myself up by leaning on my elbows, and I glanced down to see what was happening.

I saw cum trickling out my opening. At first, I thought it was precum – but there was excessively too much, and it flowed down my shaft in a slow stream. I have never felt anything like this – ever. The feeling is strange, but a good. I had no control at all; each time she hit the p-spot a little more cum flowed out of me.

"Relax Honey, let me milk you dry." I watched, as Andrea worked her fingers in me, and played with my swollen balls with her other hand. 'Oh yeah, you are nice, lose and relaxed now."

Though trembling, and on the edge of delirium from pleasure I manage to blurt out, "This feels amazing." I could feel Andrea's knuckles hitting against my ass cheeks every time she trust her fingers inside of me. My cum was now flowing almost continuously. I fell back on to the bed and closed my eyes. I could feel Andrea' mouth work back over the head of my cock and slurp away at the oozing cum.

I don't know if I am cumming or finished cumming or getting close to orgasm. It all feels so incredible, I continued to leak my juices for several more minutes as Andrea continued to plunge away at my ass and work and suck my cock. I could not control the flow – Andrea was in charge. I felt, as though I was experiencing one long orgasm, milder than a "normal orgasm" but 100 times as long.

After what seemed like a month of Sundays, Andrea whispered, "I think I will let you finish. Are you ready?"

Drenched in sweat, my heart racing, my head

about to explode and all I could say was, "Yes…yes."

Andrea dive-bombed her two fingers in my ass. I could feel her rubbing my p-spot up, down and across. Using her fingers like scissors, she gently tugged at my throbbing p-spot. With her other hand, she stroked my cock hard from the top going down to my sack almost hitting me in the balls – it felt great! She could have hit me with a hammer down there and it would have felt good. Hearing the slapping sounds Andrea was making, made my cock gush more, Andrea could not even keep up slurping it all down as the cum dribbled down my shaft, over my balls and onto the sheets.

I felt the urge to explode build up inside me. Andrea removes her soft lips from my shaft – there was no way she could handle this wad. She continued to pound my shaft and balls and plow away at my ass. I saw flashes of light …

"That's it Baby, yeah … do it, let it come," Andrea instructed.

"I'm cumming, I'm cumming," my body was almost locked up with tension. I could feel Andrea pounding my ass and balls harder. "Oh my fucking god …"

A stream shot out halfway to the ceiling, then another, another – had to be seven or eight hard shots, as I clenched my teeth having experienced the most intense orgasm I have ever felt.

"Oh my God ... HOLY SHIT! That was unbelievable," Andrea screamed.

"I cumming," I gasped.

"Baby you already said that ..." Andrea whispered.

Three more ropes surged out of me ... I was finally drained.

There is a sense of bigness with the orgasm almost as if it is being pushed out from within. Very different from a regular orgasm in that it lasts a lot longer, usually has a lot more semen, and tends to involve erogenous zones other than the cock and balls. Flashes of light; toes, back, thighs tingling.

I could not sit up; I lay there half paralyzed with my eyes closed. Andrea continued to rub the head of my cock with her fingers and then rub the puddles of cum on my stomach in soft circular motions. "My gosh, I have never seen so much cum at one time." Andrea was enjoying herself, "Had enough?"

"Oh my God yes ... please stop." Andrea removed her fingers from my ass – Almost immediately my body felt like a wet noodle. I was completely spent, my body totally exhausted. Andrea removed her stranglehold on my cock, lifted her head and said, "We have to do this again."

START WITH FOREPLAY

Andrea and I spent the next few sex sessions perfecting the P-gasm Method. Up until that night, I had vaguely heard about "milking" a man's penis, but had no idea that it was a completely new world of sexual enlightenment.

I am going to teach you how to please a man. You will make him cum like never before – you are about to learn how to give a man a p-gasm.

Start with foreplay – kissing, touching, a back rub – whatever the two of you are in the mood for. Do everything you normally would do to turn him on, do not go directly to the P-gasm Method.

Foreplay is critical, in that the P-spot swells when stimulated. This is essential; you must get him going first. This is especially important the first few times you attempt P-gasms. He should be fully stimulated and the penis fully engorged with him at the point of begging and pleading for more.

STIMULATE THE P-SPOT EXTERNALLY

Once you have him in an exited state, stimulate his p-spot externally. Do this by pressing and massaging the area of skin between his balls and anus – the perineum, commonly known as the taint. (In case you don't know from Wikipedia: Taint is a term used to refer to the perineum the region of the human body between the testicles or vagina and the anus. This term has no basis in medical terminology and is often considered lewd and mildly obscene.) AKA a "chin rest" in females. Pressing against that spot, your man will feel an internal sensation unlike anything he has felt before. Not as intense as direct penile stimulation, but he is going to be like, "Whoa! What the EFF!"

Have your man lay on his back, with you lying next to him, run your hand down between his legs. Reach down past his balls; press your finger gently on the Perineum (taint). Watch his reaction – go slow, remember that more than likely he is a virgin down there. Gradually increase the pressure and tempo of your rubbing. Lean over and gently kiss the head of his cock, to help him get over any homophobia.

At this point, your rubbing of his taint area has sent sensations to his p-spot – most likely very nice, new feelings. He feels definite warmth in the pelvis area and a deep sense of pleasure. He might not even realize that it is a sexual pleasure, maybe just a new extremely pleasant sensation. After a little while of you playing with his taint, and occasionally stroking and kissing his cock, he will realize that somehow the p-spot and his cock is connected in a sexual way.

TIME TO MOVE IN

Reach over, and swab up your finger with the lube you readied for yourself earlier. I find that the index finger works best, but some people prefer the middle finger because it is the longest. You can always change or add fingers later, so begin with your index finger.

Don't plunge in - start by rubbing his new found love hole with soft, slow circular strokes. Take your time, take it slow and easy, you will be able to tell when he is ready. Accidentally, brush his asshole a couple of times. Then just rest your finger there. If he does not like it, he will let you know. If he does, then start rubbing it. Once he starts wiggling his butt hole towards your finger, you know he is ready.

If, on the other hand he is trying to squirm away, back off his hole and rub his taint, suck his nipples, tickle the head of his cock or anything else so that he gets a breather. Do not try to rush him – more than likely you will scare the crap out of him.

After a few minutes, move your fingers back to his dark star (lube up again if necessary). As before, work your finger gently around his love hole. Slowly and gently insert your finger in his rectum – I know that the excitement and the warm feel is so exquisite that you have to control yourself not to dive in – GO SLOW.

By this time, you both are probably breaking out into a sweat, and he for sure is ready for a towel, with his skin covered in goose bumps and his nipples hard as tiny pebbles. Slowly curve your finger up towards his penis.

Grope around until you feel a small swollen bump – that is the p-spot. Once you find it, do not poke or jab at the p-spot. Gently rub it in a circular, up & down or side-to-side motion. BE GENTLE.

I don't want to berate the point, but I do have to stress, that the prostate is an internal organ not a clump of nerves – take it slow and easy at first or you will have to peel him off the ceiling. After a few sessions, you will know what he likes … or hates.

Assuming you are in, at this point, his cock is sitting straight up, twitching and dribbling out a slow stream of precum. His ass will feel like a vice clamped down on your fingers. As you move your finger inside of him, you will feel his opening flutter a little, almost as if trying to suck your finger in.

After a few minutes, lean down and take his cock into your mouth. Every time you rub against the p-spot with your finger, you will feel the throbbing and expanding of his penis. Do not poke at the p-spot unless you want him to punch a hole in the back of your head. By now, he feels as if his swollen cock has expanded to three or four times its previous size (he wishes).

MILKING THE P-SPOT

The speed, intensity and direction of your rubbing of his p-spot will influence whether your man will cum in one huge orgasm, or a Ginormous extended milking over a few minutes. A long drawn out milking is hard to achieve the first time. Arouse him to the point of ejaculation while rubbing the p-spot, and then hold him there at that point of excitement. With practice, his orgasm will last for a few minutes.

You will learn how your lover reacts to your p-spot stimulation. For him, a milking does NOT feel like a normal orgasm. At first, there is a steady flow of cum, followed by incredible "ropes" followed by more flow, then more "ropes."

It is an awesome feeling, but also kind of odd, especially the first few times. He needs to point you in the right direction, what feels good, bad or whatever. You need to experiment, try different things – and practice, practice, practice.

As the two of you practice and get better with the Method he will continue to orgasm for up to an hour or more. With you nibbling, sucking, rubbing or whatever kind of penis stimulation and gently rubbing his p-spot at the same time he will continue to cum. I'm not talking about a normal three to five second orgasm, he will have a series of mini-orgasm in between a long drawn out continuous orgasm.

WORKING THE
P-GASM METHOD

The women is in control of his orgasms; you can allow him to come full on, hold his explosion back, make him dribble, or let him explode in one big violent orgasm. Once you make him dribble cum, you can continue this cycle until he begs you to stop, or until he goes into an orgasmic coma of sorts.

If the man you are with has an active job, you might want to save this activity for special events and weekends. I can guarantee that he will be sore and have a somewhat hard time walking or sitting when the next day rolls around – especially the first few times.

Make sure you start him off with plenty of foreplay before you go exploring up the dark love tube; work him with foreplay so that he is as horny as you can make him without exploding. Be patient – you are in no rush, have fun.

Vary the pressure, speed and tempo when stimulating the p-spot until you know what he likes.

The first time or two, he might want to squirt uncontrollably right away. After a few times, you both get to know how to control his excitement and get him to flow instead.

One nice side effect of the P-gasm Method is that some men may have an urge for another orgasm within minutes of their first p-gasm. It will not happen all the time and for all men, but even after an all out milking and a full, draining orgasm to top it off, the urge will still be there for more. Not like an intentional incomplete orgasm whereby you clamp down with your PC muscles, in effect shutting off the hose but completely drained mind-blowing complete ejaculation, yet the desire for a second orgasm is intense.

On the down side, some men need an extended down time because of the draining orgasm. With time and experience, this extended down time should diminish.

Sometimes it takes repeated stimulations for the man to realize the sensations as a sexual pleasure. At first, he will recognize it as a new, different sensation, but after a while, it will become sexual and pleasurable.

Sometimes putting pillows or wrapped up towels under his butt will give you better access.

Reaction to prostate stimulation like everything else to do with sex depends on many things - how long since his previous orgasm - how did he cum last time - did he cum once, twice or what - time of the month - length of time he was stimulated, etc. Stimulating his brain is almost as important as what your mouth and fingers are doing down there.

Some men need a small butt plug to help loosen him up – most experience incredible orgasms with one of those babies up their ass. Again, go to your favorite online sex toy store and shop around.

Try this. Get in the 69 position with him on top. Yeah I know, most guys like the bottom when 69ing, he will try to resist, but insist until he agrees. While working his cock with your mouth, gently insert a finger up his ass. Encourage him to play with your ass to help keep his mind a little occupied. The first time, he might not like the insertion, but once you get going with your massage and BJ he will settle in and let you do your thing.

Once you get the milking going, those sessions can last for 20 – 30 minutes or more. When the flowing starts, it can be a constant flow with a smaller than usual final climax. Will you be able to swallow it all? That is up to you. Some girls can savor and swallow every drop even though when he cums in a "normal way" they cannot handle the whole load. Some ladies can't handle the flow – it's a personal choice.

Notes

STRAP-ON SEX

Okay, did I scare the crap out of you with that headline?

This is definitely NOT for everybody, but you would be surprised at how many men are "receptive" to this type of sexual action.

Carrie and I had been fucking for a few months. We weren't exactly boyfriend and girlfriend, but we were more than fuck-buddies. We got along great, and we both loved sex. In the beginning, it was more of a physical thing. Everything about her turned me on: that full mouth, her gorgeous rack, and those legs that went on and on. She wasn't a runway model, but she was a perfect ten in my book

It helped that her sex drive was just as high as mine was. It was hard to find a chick that wanted to fuck as often as I did. Maybe I have a high sex drive, but I think it's just normal. Some weekends we would fuck as often as five or six times a day. I usually needed a break to recover but I could keep going as long as I didn't come. Her stamina matched mine, and that's all that counted.

One weekend we decided to have a marathon fuck-fest. We cancelled all other activities and planned to spend most of the weekend in bed. I could not get enough of her tight, sexy body.

Carrie was a sexy thirty-year-old brunette with dangerous curves. She was old enough to know what she wanted out of a man. Yet, she was still young enough to want to try new things. I liked that sexually curious side of her. Whenever I suggested something new, she wanted to try it.

After a quick morning shower, we were at it again. I spread her on the bed and dove between her long legs. I kissed her calves and nibbled on her inner thighs. I touched the velvety skin between her legs. She got herself waxed so she was completely bare down there. At first it took a while getting used to the look. Then I realized that I loved how smooth she felt. I could spend all day between her legs just kissing and nibbling her.

I kissed her pussy lips while she wrapped her fingers in her hair. I wanted to take my time and make sure she got off first. I teased her clit with my tongue, flicking her gently until she gasped and groaned. I knew exactly what got her off. As I licked her hot pussy, I slid a finger inside her. She was so tight and so wet.

She moaned, "Oooooh, that's so good. You get me sooooo wet."

I continued to lick her tasty pussy until she ground her hips against my mouth. I sucked her clit and fucked her with two fingers. Soon my entire hand was wet with her sweet juices.

"Oh, fuck me," she gasped. "I want your hard cock inside me."

I got on top of her and spread her pussy lips with my fingertips. With one smooth stroke, I slid inside her. She wrapped her legs around me and I fucked her with long, slow strokes. I wanted to feel every inch of her. She was wet but she still felt unbelievably tight. I reached down to squeeze her hard nipples, and she went wild.

She thrust her hips towards me, spreading her legs even wider. I fucked her hard, slamming my cock into her. She wrapped her legs around my waist and grabbed onto my ass. I filled her with my cock as she begged for more. She breathed hard against my neck and she nibbled my earlobe. I loved when she did that, and it just made me fuck her even harder.

Carrie ground her pelvis against me and shuddered. I knew she was about to come. I pressed my cock into her with hard strokes. Her back arched and I held onto her. She shook as she moaned into my ear. I grabbed her ass and pumped into her. I was ready to come, but I wanted her to come again.

She moaned and shook with orgasm. I rolled to the side and onto my back, pulling her on top of me. Her soft body collapsed on top of mine. I could feel her thighs still trembling. I let her take a breather as I stroked her silky back and legs. She looked down at me and smiled.

"You ready to come again?" I asked her.

"You haven't come yet," she said.

"I will. Eventually. I want you to get yours first." Women loved when I said stuff like that. To be honest, it wasn't exactly a line. I usually waited until a woman came a few times before I went for mine. I loved watching a woman as she went wild with orgasm.

She ground her hips slowly against me. My cock, covered with her wetness felt great. She reached down to massage my balls. They were tight because I wanted to come. Then she grinned and slipped her hand further down. I squirmed when her finger snuck close to my asshole.

"Uhhh, sweetie? What are you doing?"

"Just playing," she said with a sweet smile.

"Ok, but that area is exit only," I joked.

"It's okay," she cooed. Her wet fingertip played with my asshole, softly stroking. Her pussy felt good around my cock, but I wasn't sure about her finger.

"Relax, baby," she said. "I'll make you feel really good." She slid off my cock and kneeled between my legs. With her finger still under my balls, she took my cock in her mouth. I heard her licking off her juices, and it got me rock hard.

She swallowed my entire cock until I hit the back of her throat. I loved when she did that. I almost came right then and there, but I was able to hold back. I didn't want the blowjob to end that soon. She was an expert, and it was almost as good as fucking.

She sucked on my cock while massaging my balls with one hand. Her mouth was nice and wet, and she let her spit get my cock and balls all slick. The fingers of her other hand teased the area under my balls. When her fingertip pressed on my asshole, I didn't mind too much. Her mouth felt too good for me to stop her.

She deep-throated me while her slick finger moved against my anus. I felt her fingertip slide inside me. I thought it would hurt, but it didn't. Actually, it almost felt good. When she slid more of it inside, I thought that it did feel good. She kept her finger there while sucking hard on me.

I lifted my head up when she stopped. She had a naughty smirk on her face. She continued stroking my cock with her hand.

"I want to *fuck you*," she whispered.

"Get on top," I told her.

"Not that way," she said. "I want to fuck you." Her finger slid further inside me.

"Exit only, baby."

"I want to use a toy on you."

"What kind of toy?" I was more curious than anything else.

She practically leaped off the bed. With her tight ass bouncing, she ran to the closet and pulled out a box. She came back with a bottle of lube and a weird-looking contraption.

I eyed her new toy with suspicion. "Is that what I think it is?"

She held up a complicated leather buckle with two looping straps. A thin, short purple dildo jutted out from the front of the flat portion. If she thought she was putting that inside me, she was crazy. I pretty much lost my hard-on right then.

I sat up and shook my head. "No fucking way. I'm not gay."

"I know you're not gay. Don't be silly! Anal stimulation doesn't make you gay."

I didn't want to hear it. Even the word anal made me uncomfortable.

"I'm not gay," I repeated.

She rolled her eyes and looked at me as if I was stupid. "No one said you're gay. Enjoying what feels good does not make you gay. You're being ridiculous."

"Whatever. I don't want anything up my ass. It's not my thing. Nope." I continued to shake my head. I thought of myself as the adventurous type, but a guy had to draw the line at some point.

"Why can't you have an open mind about it? You're pretty open about other stuff."

"That's different. We weren't talking about sticking something up my butt. I'm not even 2% gay. Not even one percent."

She pouted and crossed her arms under her fantastic rack. "That's unfair. I always try the things that you want to try. I let you try anal on me."

"It's not the same thing."

"Sure it is! I didn't think I would like anal, but it felt so good. It'll feel good to you, too." She crawled closer to me and laid her hand on my thigh. "Didn't my finger feel good?"

I couldn't answer her. She slid closer and licked my neck. I shuddered as her hot lips pressed against my ear. "I promise I'll make you feel so good, baby. It's not going to hurt. I want to fuck you so bad."

I sighed as her warm hand curled around my cock. I was hard again in an instant. There was something about her that got me rock hard whenever she was around. I didn't *want* to be turned on, but I was.

"Pleeeease? I want to try this sooooo bad." She licked my earlobe while she whispered.

"I'm not into that kind of play, honey." I tried to speak clearly even though her hand felt so good on my cock. I just wanted to let her do whatever she wanted.

"I promise I'll make it up to you. If you don't like it, I'll stop anytime. Ok, baby?"

"Let's see what happens. Keep going until either I can't handle any more or you get tired" I replied.

"OK – cool. The "out word" is "uncle.""

"What is an "out" word," I asked.

"A word you say, that immediately stops all activities. Just in case you are screaming "stop, stop," but really mean "more, more." When you say "uncle" that's it – no more," Carrie explained.

I agreed that this sounded like a good plan. "Start light and work your way up," I advised.

I sighed as she stroked me with her expert hand. She gave the most amazing hand jobs, and she knew my weaknesses. I still needed to come, and she was breaking down my defenses. Maybe if I let her do it just once, she would let me try anal again. I loved how tight her asshole felt around my cock.

"Are you sure about this?" I asked.

"Yes! Just relax and trust me." She pushed me back on the bed. She motioned me to lift my hips. When I did, she slipped a pillow under my back.

I watched her put on the buckle. She slid her legs through the loops and tightened the buckle around her waist. The small dildo suddenly looked big in front of her. I gulped when she scooted closer to me.

"Not yet," she said. She kneeled between my legs and went back to sucking my dick. My balls tightened in response to her warm, wet mouth. She worked my cock like a pro, sucking and licking while massaging my balls. I relaxed and enjoyed the leisurely blowjob. She took her time tasting and sucking every inch of me. It felt so good that I didn't want her to stop.

I felt something cold and wet under my balls. I looked down to see what she was doing. She had the bottle of lube in her hand, and her fingers looked shiny and slick. Her hand disappeared and I noticed her finger pressing against the same spot. She swallowed my cock and inserted the tip of her finger in my asshole. I gasped in surprise, but it didn't hurt. I was too focused on her mouth.

"Fuck, baby. That's nice. Suck that cock." I watched her luscious lips move up and down on my shaft. She sucked my head hard before taking it all again. Her lips had a vacuum grip on my dick.

I groaned as her finger worked its way inside me. My balls were huge and needed release soon. She slid her finger slowly in and out, in and out. Once I relaxed, I had to admit that it felt amazing. Her finger touched a sensitive spot inside my ass, and it made me squirm on the bed.

"Just relax, honey," she purred. She settled herself between my legs. The pillow under my back raised my butt a few inches. She grabbed the lube and greased up the tip of the purple dildo. For a moment, I considered chickening out. I had to admit that I was curious about how she would do this. Her take-control attitude turned me on. I stroked my cock as I watched her point the strap-on towards me. I tried not to be nervous about it.

She poured more lube on her finger and got my asshole ready for her. Then she slid the round tip closer to me. The lube felt cold but her finger was nice and warm. She finger fucked me while I jacked off. Damn, my cock was so hard.

Her finger slid out, and she replaced it with the tip of the dildo. She smiled and scooted an inch forward. I felt something against my asshole. I could tell the toy itself was thin, but it was a little thicker than her finger. She guided the strap-on with one hand and stroked my hard cock with the other.

"That feels good, doesn't it?" she whispered. Her voice was all breathy like she was turned on, too.

I stared at her beautiful tits. "Does this make your pussy wet, Carrie?"

Her eyes got all round and shiny. "Oh, yes, baby. I'm so turned on right now."

"Ooooh, Carrie. Don't stop. You feel sooooo good."

She grinned and slid the tip of the dildo inside my ass. I could feel it stretch my asshole, and it entered after some pushing. I prepared myself for the pain, but there was just a slight pressure as the head slid into me. Other than that, it didn't feel weird or wrong at all. It actually made my cock even harder.

She pushed my knees back and slid another inch inside my asshole. It was tight but the lube helped. She gently rocked back and forth on her heels, just sliding the tip in and out of my ass. She rubbed more lube on her hand and covered my cock with it. She grabbed hard and stroked me with quick jerks, her hand moving up and down like a piston.

"Does it hurt, baby?" she asked in a husky voice.

"No. It feels good. Almost too good."

"That's what I like to hear." She rocked her hips until she was fucking me. I couldn't believe that a hot sexy woman was actually fucking me. It felt good, and it was total mind-fuck. I had to admit that I enjoyed every minute of it. She looked down at me with a sexy, naughty grin on her face. She got off on the power trip, and so did I.

"Doesn't it feel good? Doesn't it feel good to be fucked like this?"

"Ooooh, Carrie. You're so good. God, don't stop. Aaaaaaah, fuck!"

I felt her toy fill me up. My balls were so tight that it was almost painful. Her hand tugged at my dick until I thought I would explode. She made little grunts as she fucked me with her strap-on. Her hips moved in time with her lube-covered hand. First with the long, slow strokes, then in a faster rhythm. She fucked me like she knew exactly what she was doing. It was too much at once.

"Oooooh, Carrie! I'm so close! I'm going to come!"

Just as I was about to come, she pushed the dildo deeper. My cock jerked wildly in her hand and shot come all over her breasts and neck. My come shot straight up in the air. There was just so much of it. Some of it even reached her luscious lips. I watched her tongue lick off my hot seed. I've never come so hard in my life.

The strap-on slid out of me and she hopped off the bed. She returned with a warm, damp towel and helped clean the lube off me. I was too spent to help her. All I could do was lay on my back and stare at her sexy body. I reached between her legs to touch her moist pussy.

"You're so wet, baby." I touched her swollen pussy lips. I hadn't even fucked her yet, and she was already so wet.

"I know. You turned me on so much."

"Did you really like that?"

"I enjoyed it as much as you did." She winked.

Maybe not. I may have enjoyed it more than she did. But I didn't have to tell her that. As soon as I recovered, I'd show her how much I enjoyed myself.

Say Hello to Flo

Flo, a petite brunette with a cute little body and I were at her house partying. At the time, we had only been going out for a very short time, and had just started to have sex on a regular basis.

We both had a few beers, and were feeling good. "Have you ever had a p-gasm?" Flo asked.

"P-gasm?" I asked, knowing what she was talking about and just waiting for her reaction. I have had the pleasure of a p-gasm, but Flo and I had never discussed p-gasms before.

"P-gasms," She repeated. "You know, a p-spot stimulated orgasm," Flo explained.

I tried to keep a blank face, hoping that she would reveal more information. Flo and I had been going out for about a month, and our relationship was starting to become serious and I wanted to know where she was going with this.

I snuggled closer to her, rested my head on her soft shoulder, inhaled her sweet scent. "What do you think?" Flo asked with a teasing voice that made her smile. "You want to give it a try?"

Flo pulled me closer to her, and drew her mouth close to mine. Her soft lips pressed hard against mine, and my tongue parted her lips as I explored her silky mouth.

Her nipples poked out from her t-shirt. I pinched them playfully, causing Flo to let out a soft moan. I peeled away her shirt. Her bra concealed her big beautiful breasts. Flo reached back, undid the snap and let me get a glimpse of her milky white tits. Her bra straps slipped off her shoulders and the silky bra fell to the floor.

By now my engorged dick was trying to tear through my jeans. Flo reached down between my legs "You have quite the bulge," Flo giggled, struggling to get the zipper to slide down over my expanded manhood. Finally, she slipped my jeans down to my ankles and exclaimed, "Ooh, you're a tighty whitey guy. Great ass! I don't know what I like better, the outline of your cock in those tight pants, or your butt." Flo yanked on the elastic band to get a peek inside before sliding them down my legs and onto the ground.

"OK, enough of this," Flo commanded, "Let's move to your bedroom." Once there, Flo pushes me onto the bed and removes any excess clothing from me. Once I was completely undressed, Flo tossed aside the bed comforter to reveal two black straps fastened lengthwise across the top of the mattress.

"Oh my GOD," I thought to myself, "What the fuck is she up to?" I was a little scared, but man was I excited, my cock throbbing with anticipation.

"Get on the bed – face down," Flo commanded. She fastened each of my wrists with the straps. I was worried, but the fear was nothing compared to my excitement. She grabbed her still warm pantyhose, and wrapped them securely around the base of my shaft and around my balls.

With me on my all fours, Flow positioned herself under my cock and with her juicy red lips greedily played with the head of my cock. She ran her warm tongue up and down and around my shaft and balls. "This was unbelievable," I thought to myself.

Flo slid out from under me and asked, "I bet you like it in the ass – don't you?" My heart nearly stopped. I watched as Flo put on a harness with a dildo attached. She applied a generous amount of lube on her new-found manhood and positioned herself behind me. Slowly she sunk that thing into me. It was the oddest feeling I ever felt, yet Flo knew exactly where to hit the p-spot.

At first, she did it slowly, very slowly, and it didn't hurt as much as I thought it might have. Flo was very talented with that dildo, almost as if it was real. Eventually she began to pound away at me with her tits flapping across my back. Every time she hit the p-spot, my cock gushed out cum – the bed was soaked already, and I didn't even cum yet.

Every now and then between thrusts, Flo would reach between my legs and give my cock a few violent strokes. I was about to lose it, "I'm gonna cummm ..."

"In my mouth, Baby"

She works her way down on her back between my legs and begins to suck me off. She works a finger into my anus and violently finger fucks me, hitting the p-spot constantly. I can't take it and my body lets go. I have an intense incredible orgasm. I feel the cum fly out of my penis into her waiting mouth. Flo gags with my fierce eruption, but the trooper she is, not a drop hits the mattress.

MILKING &
A HUMMER

From the moment I met her, I recognized that Janet was the sexually adventurous type. She had that confident, slightly aggressive vibe about her. It was in the way she touched my arm, shoulder, and later my upper thigh. I liked a woman who knew what she wanted, and I could tell that she wanted me.

I met her the first time on a Wednesday night. I didn't plan to meet anyone that night. It was my buddy's idea to go to the new bar called The Velvet, but I wasn't too interested. I figured it would be one of those typical new bars with watered-down, expensive drinks and unnecessary cover charge. My friend Greg had just been dumped by his girlfriend, and he needed cheering up. I was the designated wing man.

I didn't mind being the wing man. I just ended things with a fuck buddy who wanted more, and I wasn't ready to get back in the game. Not yet. It would take a special woman to coax me back out of my shell.

By midnight I had a nice buzz going, and Greg worked his natural charm on a bubbly brunette with a fantastic rack. He bet me that they were natural C-cups, and he was determined to find out the truth. Greg didn't need a wingman anymore.

"Is this seat taken?"

I looked up and saw the most amazing pair of green eyes. I'm not one to notice a woman's eyes first. That's how amazing they were. I barely managed to smile and said, "Nope, it's all yours."

She flashed a grin full of pearly, straight teeth. "Thanks. I'm Janet."

We exchanged the typical small talk. I tried not to stare at her cleavage that practically spilled out of her low-cut top. She made it hard because she leaned over a lot. She was a pretty brunette with a natural tan and long hair. She had curves in all the right places, and she had a nice ass for someone so thin.

From her lean arms and toned stomach, she seemed the type that either spent a lot of time at the gym or on the beach. When she laughed, she tossed her head back to give me a good look at her nice rack. I didn't know what I liked better: her gorgeous body or her cute face.

Usually I'm clueless when a woman flirts with me. Hey, I'm a guy --- I'm bad with reading the signs. It was a good thing that Janet's signals were more obvious. As the conversation went on, her hands became a little friendlier. First, she touched my thighs as she talked. Eventually her hand was just inches away from my package. I hoped she didn't notice the obvious bulge.

I moved her shirt up a little so I could touch the small of her back. "Is it okay if I touch you here?"

She giggled and tossed her hair again. The simple gesture got me hard already. "I don't mind."

"Good." Her skin felt warm and soft.

She caressed my forearm. "You know what? I've been told that I'm a fabulous kisser."

I wasn't an idiot. I wasn't going to let that slide. "Really? Well, why don't I be the judge of that?" It was a cheesy line, and I didn't expect it to work. I was buzzed, horny, and decided to give it a chance.

Janet smiled and leaned towards me for the most amazing kiss. Her full lips were soft and tender. She nibbled on my lower lip before she stuck her hot tongue in my mouth. I grabbed around the waist and pulled her closer. Close enough to rub my hard-on against her. That seemed to excite her even more. I felt her moan deep in her throat, and I couldn't wait to hear more of that sexy moaning.

She paused for a breather. "Maybe we should get out of here before we get arrested for public indecency?"

"You read my mind." I nodded to Greg as we left the bar.

It was a short cab ride to her apartment. We kissed and petted in the back seat like we were two college kids again. Her breasts felt soft and natural. I snuck my hand under shirt and played with her hardening nipples. She writhed when I rolled her nipple under my fingers. I gave her a playful pinch, and she practically jumped in my lap. I thought I was one lucky bastard when her hand went straight for my cock.

With a devious smile, she whispered, "I have an oral fixation."

I tried not to look surprised. Instead I grinned. "Lucky me."

Janet was even more aggressive when we entered her apartment. I really was lucky that night. She had my pants down before I made it to her sofa. I pulled her shirt and bra off and went straight for those delicious tits. She moaned as I sucked and kissed her breasts, teasing her nipples with my tongue.

I touched the front of her soaking wet panties. I cupped her mound, rubbing my palm against her clit. She made sexy sounds and writhed against my hand. I moved her panties out of the way and touched her wet pussy. She was ready for a nice, hard fuck.

Before I could do anything else, she dropped to her knees and pulled down my pants. My cock strained against my boxer-briefs as she put her mouth against me. I guess she wanted a blowjob more than sex. I didn't have a problem with that.

She teased me with her mouth, rubbing her lips over my crotch and breathing hard against me. Her hot breath made my dick throb. Her lips hadn't even touched my cock, and I was harder than I'd ever been. She definitely had the magic touch.

"That feels so good," I groaned.

"I know what feels even better." She pulled down my underwear and swallowed my dick all the way to my balls. She didn't even hesitate. She just took my dick until I hit the back of her throat. She was right about having an oral fixation.

"Holy shit. You're an expert, baby." I caressed her soft hair as she slid my cock in and out of her mouth. She paused to stroke the shaft and lick my head. I gazed down into her sparkling green eyes. I saw the smile on her face as she sucked me like she couldn't get enough of me. I didn't want to come yet, but she made it difficult to hold back.

She stopped and said, "Want to take it to the bedroom?"

I couldn't believe how sexy she was. It really was my lucky night. "I'm all yours, beautiful."

I removed the rest of my clothes and joined her in the bedroom. I ran my hands all over her gorgeous body. She was even hotter than I thought she would be. Her natural C-cups were full and bouncy. Her shaved pussy looked juicy and inviting. When I reached for her, she stopped me. "I'm not done with my oral fixation yet."

I laughed. "Good to know."

"Lay down on the bed."

She was assertive, and I liked that about her. My dick sprang straight in the air as she crawled between my legs. She leaned down to take my cock in her mouth again. I noticed she had something in her hand, but I was too distracted to comment on it. All I could think about was her mouth milking my cock. She sucked hard like she wanted my hot come right away.

"Damn, girl, that feels so fucking good." I ran my fingers through her thick hair and watched her work my dick.

She moaned around my cock and stared into my eyes. The eye contact drove me wild. I loved when chicks did that. I watched as she slid her tongue all over my shaft and then up and down the sides of my cock. She used her hand to stroke my shaft while sucking hard on the head. She sat back and admired the way my cock glistened.

She licked her hand and stroked me, wrapping her long fingers around me. She bent forward and wrapped her lips around my cock. Her mouth drove me wild. From time to time, she changed her movements from deep, long strokes to short, quick sucks.

I closed my eyes and enjoyed her tongue. I groaned as she massaged my balls. When her finger got a little too close to my asshole, I almost jumped out of my skin.

"Hold on, sexy," I said.

She ignored me and rubbed my asshole with a tender finger. I froze for a second until I realized that she was doing that on purpose. I scooted up the bed and out of her reach.

"I don't think so," I said. The blowjob was phenomenal, but this was more than I bargained for.

She sat back on her heels and looked at me. "What's the big deal? I promise that it feels really good."

"It's uncomfortable. I'm not down with that."

"I really want to milk you. It will feel so good."

"Milk me?"

She looked surprised. "Haven't you ever heard of that?"

I shook my head.

"It's when I give you a blowjob while stimulating your prostate."

It sounded weird. "Stimulating with what?"

"My finger. Don't worry. I have lube." She said it in a no-nonsense tone like it wasn't a big deal. Like it was something she did all the time.

I debated getting off the bed. She was damn hot, but I wasn't sure about that kind of thing. "I'm not into that."

She rolled her eyes. "Did you know that your prostate is an erogenous zone?"

"What?" I didn't know what she was talking about.

"Think of the prostate as the male G-spot. You have all sorts of nerve endings in there." She cupped my balls as she talked. "Prostate stimulation feels good for men. Combine that with a blowjob, and it's mind-blowing." She gave me a knowing look. "Trust me. You'll thank me afterwards."

I concentrated on the way her soft hand felt. She definitely knew how to keep me hard. Still I was uncertain. "I'm not sure I want anything up my ass."

"It doesn't make you gay," she said. "A lot of straight guys are missing out on an amazing experience." She spit on her hand and stroked my cock as she talked. I was hard as a rock and wanted her mouth on me again.

"You want to suck that again?"

She gave me a sly grin. "Only if you let me milk you."

Damn her. She knew I couldn't say no. "We'll try it, but I don't know if I'll like it."

"Trust me," she said. "Lay back. Relax. Let me do all the work."

"What have you got there?"

She held up a clear plastic bottle. "Lube."

I closed my eyes and tried to relax. It wasn't easy until I felt her hot mouth envelop my cock. "Fuck. That's so good."

She stopped to say, "It gets even better."

I tensed up when I felt her slick finger press against my anus. I concentrated on how her mouth felt and tried to relax. Her lubed fingertip slipped under my balls and went back to my ass. I had to admit that it didn't feel bad. I was harder than before.

Her lips moved up and down on my shaft. My cock was hard and wet from her mouth. When she slipped her fingertip inside my ass, it didn't feel as weird as I thought it would. I was afraid that she'd fuck me with her finger, but she just kept it there while she sucked me.

I groaned as she wrapped her mouth around my dick. She started to take it deeper and deeper. At the same time, her lubed finger slid further inside my asshole. She slowly slid the tip of her finger in and out. Once I relaxed, it started to feel good. Really good.

"Fuck, Janet. That feels incredible."

She laughed with my dick in her mouth. It sounded more like a mumble. Her finger slid in deeper, and I jumped when she pressed it inside me. I could feel her fingertip against a particular spot. The sensations sent shockwaves through me. My balls got tight, and I wanted to come right then.

She stopped long enough to say, "Not yet. Don't come."

I held on as she rubbed her finger inside me. I assumed that she found my prostate gland. I don't know what she found, but I know she had the magic touch. Her finger moved slow and gentle as her mouth bobbed up and down on my cock. She stroked me on the inside until my hips started thrusting towards her mouth. I couldn't help it. The combined sensations drove me crazy.

"Damn, don't stop, baby. Don't stop!"

I felt her finger slid deeper and press harder against that same spot. She rubbed with a little more pressure and I thought my cock would explode. Her finger moved faster until I fucked her mouth with abandon. She sucked the head of my cock as she moved her finger in and out of me. I couldn't believe that I was letting her finger fuck my ass. I couldn't believe that I didn't mind. Hell, I fucking loved it.

"Ah, fuck! Oh, fuck…that feels so damn good. Oh my god, you're so fucking good."

My balls felt huge, and I knew I was going to come hard. I wanted the feeling to last as long as possible. She took my cock deep into her mouth and continued to massage that spot inside my ass. She increased the pressure inside me, rubbing her fingertip back and forth. I didn't want her to stop. I didn't want to come, but I knew I couldn't hold back any longer.

"Oh my god, Janet. I'm going to come. I want to come inside that sweet mouth."

She responded by sucking harder. Her lips were so tight around my rock-hard cock. She licked and sucked me with abandon. I could tell that this was turning her on, too. I could see it in the way she practically gagged on my cock. I could tell that she loved to deep throat. Her finger continued to press and rub against that special spot. I wanted to come so bad, but I couldn't get enough.

"Can I come in your mouth, baby? I'm going to come so hard for you. Damn, that's soooo good."

She moaned around my cock. It sounded like "Mmmmmm." She slipped her finger further inside my ass. Not too deep but I could feel more of her. And that was enough to set me off.

"Oooooooh, fuck!"

I groaned as I shot my come into her delicious mouth. She sucked me greedily, swallowing my hot seed. I thrust my cock between her lips, my hips moving up and down. It was the longest orgasm I ever had. I almost thought that I couldn't stop coming. I emptied my balls deep into her mouth. She sucked harder, milking my cock out of every last drop.

"Holy shit," I said when I could finally catch my breath. "Damn. Just damn."

She sat back and wiped her lips demurely. "How was that?"

"That was the most intense orgasm I've ever had."

Her smile glowed. "I told you it would feel really good."

I almost blushed when I thought about it. Here I was with this hot chick who had her finger up my ass. It was insane. I couldn't believe that I let anyone try that, but I was glad that I did.

"I like watching a man get off like that," she said. "There's nothing weird or wrong about it. It feels really good for the guy, and I like doing it."

"Good to know." I was spent. All I could do was lay back and stare at the ceiling. What an incredible experience. I was so lucky to have run into someone who was so sexually adventurous. I never imagined that a prostate massage would feel so great. I wondered about the other tricks she had up her sleeve.

MILKING A MAN AND ORGASM DENIAL

The following was not written by me – I couldn't make this up -I have no experience in this arena of the milking process – way over my head.

Milking a man can be used as a tool to control a man – denial of orgasmic release can be a powerful weapon used by a Dominatrix.

What follows is testimony from an experienced male submissive, courtesy LongSlowPlays telling of the complex joy of his being enslaved by his Mistress thru orgasm denial, milking, and deep rectal manipulation:

"As far as the milking, I am not only getting used to this, but I actually crave it more than any other thing. It used to take longer but now I find that once the massaging starts, my penis starts to drip and ooze right away. I love the slow oozing, I love the taste, I love being kept open beneath her.

What is male milking, you ask? Some might think it is the repeated forced masturbation of the male slave to the point of his finally not being able to ejaculate. Some think it is the teasing and stimulation right up to the point of ejaculation, but with no actual release – taking him to the edge over and over, driving him batty with the denial of ultimate release. While such methods do insure a certain modicum of control, the most effective technique goes much deeper into his being.

True milking actually denies the slave the one thing he truly loves to do the most: to explode his essence in a wild and utterly incapacitating explosive release. And this denial is achieved through the skillful violation up into his most vulnerable orifice.

True milking is the controlled stimulation of the male sub's prostate gland, causing the non-eruptive discharge of his semen ... "discharge" and "leakage" instead of spurted ejaculation.

Because discharge is not orgasmic like an ejaculation, but more of a constant maddening oozing and draining of his essence. She prevents him from his release, holding him at a point where her purposes are the only ones that matter. He is well stimulated, to be sure, but the intensity is so well controlled by her that he becomes his Lady's total slave.

This is denial, but with a critical difference: his deepest inner sexuality is manipulated to the point that enslavement to her wishes is his only release, is what binds him enduringly and without reservation to thorough and endlessly wholehearted pleasuring of his Lady.

The prostate is a small gland in men, felt approximately three inches up inside the rectum, surrounding the neck of the bladder and urethra. Its primary function is to contribute to seminal fluid.

Milking is the deep and continual massaging of the prostate and surrounding area. Continual massaging of his prostate forces the slow release of his semen down through his urethra to his penis. This deep rectal forcing of his fluids is so spellbinding to him that it eventually and irrevocably makes him her sexual slave.

The massaging can be by fingers, or an object like a dildo. Fingers are the best for stimulation but a dildo will also work quite well and aids greatly in the humbling loss of control.

Lengthy practice will assure the acquiring of the best technique for optimum dildo control and consequent anal enslavement of the male. Regular size vibrating dildos of about 6-8 inches in length are best. A ribbed dildo is particularly effective.

As stated earlier, unlike masturbation, which results in an explosive release (ejaculation), massaging of the prostate to the point of milking is neither explosive nor as acutely ecstatic for him.

Again, massaging the prostate and milking the slave is a slow process that results in the draining of his essence as well as the draining away of his will to resist his Lady. It is hypnotically pleasurable but nowhere near the acute pleasure of cumming by jerking-off, or by being jerked off.

During milking, the cum oozes out in slow drips and there is no explosive ejaculation.

To aid in the milking, grasp the base of the penis and squeeze the juices out while massaging the prostate.

These expressed juices can be simultaneously smeared around his lips and nose while he is being probed with dildo or strap-on, to aid greatly in the re-conditioning process.

When being used anally via dildo, to get the best stimulation to his prostate he must also assist her by working the dildo against his prostate, arching and bending into its pressures.

He will be more than eager to do this, grinding his hips. With practice he will become most uninhibited in his gyrations. So his Lady not only fucks him, but he fucks himself for her. He becomes her dancing erotic puppet at the end of her control.

Another thing about milking is that the slow drippings of his cum always leave him only partially satisfied, and constantly sexually frustrated ... he has a constant feeling of being on the verge of cumming so he keeps grinding and massaging, or wanting his prostate to be massaged, in the hopes of actually cumming.

Blinded by the spell of her manipulatory invasions, he turns, moans and is helpless. This is great for her, because right after a typical slave cums, he loses a lot of his submissiveness, and with a reduced feeling of submissiveness, the Lady also loses some of her control.

Not so with milking: the slave is never fully sexually satisfied so he remains sexually frustrated, submissive, obedient and attentive. He will beg and weep and beseech his Lady to keep fucking him so he can get closer and closer to his release. Yet it keeps him on the edge of his ejaculation, without that critical orgasmic release.

His experience is a lot like what his Lady sometimes feels during clitoral stimulation from hand massaging, or from oral service, or from fucking, but incompletely so - if such stimulation continues and is done properly, his Lady can climax in a very strong manner, similar to when a male ejaculates.

Not so with milking, since he remains on the edge throughout the milking, however long she may wish to prolong it. This makes him crave more and more stimulation, hoping he will be allowed a strong and final orgasm. The cruel and delightful truth is that it never comes, not for him. She can keep him willingly maddened indefinitely, subject to whatever erotic whims she demands.

What happens is the male becomes more eager to please her and to feel the extremes of her manipulation. Instead of the orgasmic release of cum, only those drips of cum ooze out... with ease she gets him to lick his own forced dribbles from her hand, addicting him to the juice she forces out of him – since he is constantly draining and constantly kept from a full-blown ejaculation.

The slave then comes to crave this taste of himself and this state of affairs and becomes conditioned to these subtle but extraordinary sensations, knowing it's the only way to please her. So his Lady, thru teasing, orgasm denial, and milking, conditions him endlessly, and she gets him to love being fucked up the ass (and to finding his penis relatively useless, except for peeing and dripping cum ... it's entirely up to Her!).

She can get him to love drinking his own essences and, through her dildo fucking him constantly, love to be taken anally over and over for long periods of time. She can settle over his face with her own hips as she continues to grind her dildo against his inner organ, forcing him to pleasure both her clit and asshole with his nose and lips and tongue as long as she wishes, rubbing herself over his upturned head exhaustingly, thru the repeated multiple orgasms she will be able to give herself.

Not exactly face-sitting, this is more like face fucking - An ideal posture of worship for the male and for the female alike. And if the Lady is one who particularly enjoys having her the rim of her anal sphincter tongue-fucked, she will be able to indulge herself in this pleasure indefinitely. He will beg her not to stop fucking him, burying his tongue repeatedly.

He becomes her lap dog forever, if that's what she wants . . . he will deny her nothing. His upturned cheeks are hers for the taking, whenever and however and for as long as she needs. Her only limit will be her own ongoing imagination and physical stamina.

She paces herself by alternating deep rectal churning with other activities, gradually reshaping the contours of his libidinous nature to her own lust. She eventually gets his conditioning to the point of making him bow to her wishes. With no actual stimulation of his penis at all, simply through touching the vibrating head of her dildo to his pucker, or even just by saying it -- a whispered promise that she's going to fuck him will have him on his knees instantly, his happy, eager face upturned. Or anything else upturned. Lady's Choice!

Because the male's truest submissive nature is most clearly revealed while he is in a state of sexual frustration, it's best to persist with this particular method of domination at all times. To keep him in a state of total need and uninhibited willingness to please her is the goal. And, as explained above, milking is what accomplishes this, beyond any other technique at her disposal."

Holy crap – that is some heavy shit. As I said before, the preceding was not my story – that was written by a submissive that loves to get his P-spot milked. Is he happy? Who knows.

Hope this dude has a real life also.

Curing Your Minuteman

I don't usually discuss this subject directly with a woman, but oftentimes premature ejaculation is a nightmare for an otherwise successful relationship.

In other words … what if he comes too fast to get you off, and leaves you sexually frustrated and angry towards him.

This is the curse of many a man and can spell certain doom in your quest for milking the male species. But it doesn't have to be that way. You can help by gently encouraging him to read the following advice.

Read this and do the exercises EVERY DAY.

There are several ways for you to stave off an unwanted climax. The most popular and overused way is to think about baseball. This is hackneyed sitcom fodder but it might work for some of you. The problem, though, is that while you're imagining baseball, you're subconsciously realizing that you're thinking about baseball because you've got this hot, naked bitch under you.

All of a sudden, the image of A-Rod will do nothing to keep a lid on your syringe (no offense there A-Rod). You'll think about baseball and then you'll think about ballpark dogs. Next you'll think about buns and you'll be right there in the same pickle.

Imagining something else CAN work in some instances, though. Try thinking about your grandmother when you feel like you're about to come. If that doesn't work, think about your grandmother sucking your grandfather's dick. If that doesn't work, think about your mom eating out your grandmother. Just keep thinking about family members and you should be able to stave off the inevitable for a little longer.

Another great trick is to think about the real world. If you have a pressing deadline at work, for instance, just thinking about it for a few seconds can allow you to worry just enough to take your mind off the action and keep thrusting for a bit longer. If you owe somebody money and they're particularly angry about it, imagine the beating you'll receive in the near future. You get the idea.

Another great tip involves your…well…tip. Pulling out and pinching your dickhead with a thumb on the top and a finger on the bottom can help keep you from coming. Do this discreetly, when changing positions or something similar. Squeezing your balls fairly hard works too, but it isn't for everyone. Flicking the balls is a similar trick that works well for some people, and not as well for others.

I know it's a little bit of a sissy-man position, but being on the bottom works in staving off an on-coming orgasm. If you're on top and you feel like you're about to blow your load, try flipping over and putting her on top.

Ever hear of Kegels?

Kegels exercises are working out the muscles that you contract when you hold your piss in because you don't want to stop at that gas station where those cretins are hanging out. They are also the same muscles that keep you from coming.

Try it now. Act like you want to stop your piss. Feel that contraction? Those are your PC muscles, which stand for pubococcygeus. To master when and where you shoot your scrotal soda your PC muscles need a workout.

So how do you strengthen these muscles?

It's easy and far more entertaining than doing crunches. Do these exercises **every day for the rest of your life**. Within a couple of weeks, you'll notice a marked difference in your ability to contain your penis Pepsi from shooting out at inopportune moments.

You can do these exercises anywhere: while driving; waiting in line at the bank; waiting in line at the grocery store; do them while at work, etc. Once you are skilled at Kegel exercises, you should be able to do them without anyone else knowing what you are doing.

Go to your local adult shop and pick up a few cock rings. They don't have to be the expensive type (no metal) – a couple of bucks at most. The "o-rings" at Home Depot work well also. Buy a few different sizes so that you can get the right inside diameter. Cock rings engorge your penis by stopping the blood flow out of your cock. Cock rings also help prevent premature ejaculation. As an added bonus, cock rings give your dick a nice fat, chubby look. They don't make your cock any longer, but a properly fit cock ring will make your meat "girthier."

A Kegel exercise program along with wearing a cock ring is the most powerful method for ending embarrassing premature ejaculation. You'll literally be able to "turn off the hose" – very POWERFUL.

PC Muscles – Kegels For Men

Here's a simple set of exercises that can bring back a firmer erection, create mind-blowing orgasms and give you the ability to "turn off the hose". Strong PC muscles give you the ability to stop the flow of ejaculate during orgasm, thereby delaying and prolonging your fun. When you finally do ejaculate, you might splatter the headboard behind you.

To find your PC muscle, start to urinate then stop in midstream. If you have trouble stopping the flow of urine, you probably also have weak orgasms and premature ejaculation.

Do not exercise while urinating.

PC clamps: squeeze and release, start by holding for five seconds and then gradually increase the time. Start with "sets" of ten, and build up to sets of 100 or more. Do these every day for the rest of your life. This is a great exercise while you are driving or standing on line at the grocery store.

Long squeeze: Hold your PC muscle compressed tight for a count of twenty. Build up the strength to 30 or 50 count.

Slow squeeze: Tighten the PC muscle as slowly as you possibly can – repeat as often as you can.

You can do these exercises anywhere and at any time, there is absolutely no excuse to neglect your exercises. No one will know that you are squeezing, unless of course you keep smiling like a dumb ass while doing them, thinking about the next WT session.

PC Muscles – Kegels for Women

Kegel exercises were originally created to help women strengthen their PC muscles to help stop urinary incontinence after childbirth, when the PC muscle has been stretched out. The Kegel exercise turns out, has sexual benefits also.

There are three reasons she should do her Kegel exercises.

First, a strong PC muscle will help her overcome the "have to pee" feeling during the G-gasm Method we discussed briefly at the beginning of this book.

Second, when the PC muscle is stretched out, less of the vagina and G-spot area is in direct contact with the penis and therefore receives less stimulation – less fun for her and you.

Thirdly, a well-toned PC muscle will give her a powerful ejaculation. Keep the PC muscle exercised with Kegels – she will have greater blood flow to the area, and the greater ability to become aroused and feel sexual pleasure.

The great thing about doing Kegel exercises is that no one knows you are doing them. While you can do all sorts of variations, the basic female Kegel exercises are:

Contract your PC muscles. Hold initially for a count of five; build up gradually to a count of twenty. Repeat ten times and practice daily. Like with all muscles you are better off building the PC muscle slowly and regularly.

LETTERS

Got to say that this really works. Gave my man a BJ last night and I did the p-massage, probed his prostate and talk about COME! I didn't think he was going to quit. This lasted for a good hour before he couldn't handle it anymore. Will definitely be doing this more often. Thanks a bunch for introducing this to us.

Kathy P. – New York, NY

Last night my girl told me if she'd been born a man she would be gay. She seduced me, not for regular first time sex but.....mmm....she wanted to get my pants down so she could get at my ass.

John G. – Reno, NV

My wife had me go down on all fours, she massaged my prostrate while a puddle built up on the tile floor. After a while she did me with a dildo, talking me through pushing and tightening on it until I had what felt like an internal orgasm - never felt that before.

Nick I. – LA, CA

Go to:

BonniesGang.com

Sign-up for our newsletter,

and receive your bonus report:

Hot and Heavy

Top Five Myths about the Female Orgasm

CPSIA information can be obtained
at www.ICGtesting.com
Printed in the USA
FFOW02n0648260917
40381FF